HIGH BLOOD PRESSURE COOKBOOK

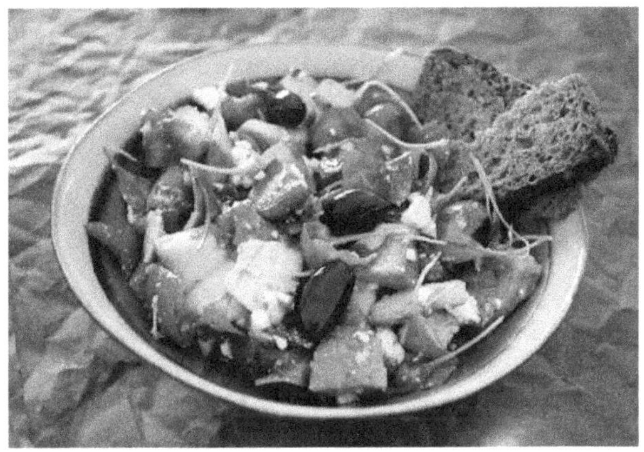

DR. JESSICA SMITH

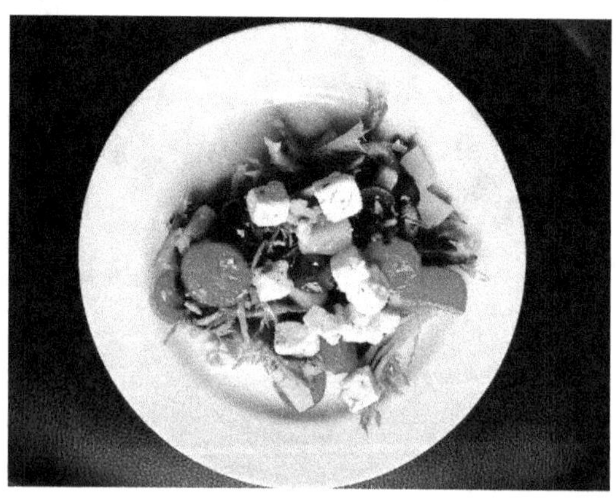

TABLE OF CONTENTS

CHAPTER ONE

How to Use this Cookbook

Familiarize Yourself with the Cookbook:

Start by flipping through the High Blood Pressure Cookbook to get an overview of the recipes and the variety of meals it offers.

Read the Introduction and Guidelines:

Pay close attention to the cookbook's introduction. Look for guidelines, tips, and recommendations related to managing high blood pressure through diet.

Understand Portion Sizes:

Take note of recommended portion sizes for different recipes. Managing portion control is crucial for maintaining a balanced diet, especially for individuals dealing with high blood pressure.

Identify Key Ingredients:

Identify key ingredients that are known for their blood pressure-friendly properties, such as potassium-rich foods, lean proteins, whole grains, and heart-healthy fats.

Meal Planning:

Plan your meals for the week based on the cookbook's recipes. Consider including a variety of dishes to ensure a balanced and nutritious diet.

Check for Nutritional Information:

Refer to the nutritional information provided for each recipe. Look for details like sodium content, as monitoring sodium intake is crucial for managing high blood pressure.

Experiment with Flavorful Herbs and Spices:

Embrace the cookbook's recommendations for using herbs and spices to add flavor without relying heavily on salt. Experiment with different combinations to enhance the taste of your dishes.

Prepare Shopping Lists: Before heading to the grocery store, make a shopping list based on the recipes you've chosen. This ensures you have all the necessary ingredients at hand and reduces the temptation to buy unhealthy options.

Follow the Cooking Instructions: When preparing meals, carefully follow the cooking instructions provided in the cookbook. Pay attention to cooking methods that promote heart health, such as grilling, baking, steaming, and sautéing with healthy oils.

Monitor Your Blood Pressure:

As you incorporate recipes from the High Blood Pressure Cookbook into your diet, regularly monitor your blood pressure levels. Keep track of any positive changes and consult with your healthcare provider if needed.

Understanding High Blood Pressure Cookbook

Understanding this High Blood Pressure Cookbook is a crucial step toward managing hypertension through mindful and heart-healthy eating.

This cookbook is a comprehensive guide that goes beyond providing recipes; it serves as a roadmap for individuals seeking to adopt a dietary approach to control and prevent high blood pressure.

Within its pages, you'll find a wealth of information on ingredients known for their positive impact on blood pressure.

This cookbook emphasizes the inclusion of potassium-rich foods, lean proteins, whole grains, and heart-healthy fats, all of which play pivotal roles in maintaining cardiovascular health.

It encourages readers to explore the use of flavorful herbs and spices as alternatives to excessive salt, promoting a culinary experience that is both health-conscious and satisfying.

Furthermore, this cookbook serves as a practical tool for meal planning and preparation. With carefully curated recipes and nutritional information accompanying each dish, individuals can easily create well-balanced and delicious meals.

By following the cooking instructions and embracing the cookbook's guidance, users can embark on a journey toward improved heart health, making informed dietary choices that contribute to overall well-being.

Principles of High Blood Pressure Cookbook

The principles of this high blood pressure cookbook revolve around promoting heart-healthy eating habits to manage and prevent hypertension.

First and foremost, this cookbook emphasizes a reduction in sodium intake, as excessive salt consumption is a major contributor to elevated blood pressure.

It encourages the use of herbs, spices, and other flavor-enhancing ingredients to replace salt and maintain the taste of the dishes.

Furthermore, this cookbook prioritizes a diet rich in fruits and vegetables, which are excellent sources of potassium, a mineral known for its blood pressure-lowering effects.

Whole grains, lean proteins, and healthy fats are also key components, ensuring a balanced and nutritious approach to meals. Portion control is emphasized to manage calorie intake and maintain a healthy weight, another crucial factor in blood pressure management.

This cookbook promotes cooking techniques that retain nutrients while minimizing the use of unhealthy fats and oils. Emphasis is placed on incorporating heart-healthy oils, such as olive oil, and limiting saturated and trans fats. Additionally, the recipes are designed to include foods high in magnesium and calcium, which play roles in blood pressure regulation.

Benefits of High Blood Pressure Cookbook

This high blood pressure cookbook offers a multitude of benefits for individuals seeking to manage and improve their cardiovascular health. Firstly, this cookbook provide a structured and accessible guide for creating meals that prioritize ingredients known to lower blood pressure.

By focusing on nutrient-dense foods like fruits, vegetables, and whole grains, this cookbook facilitate a balanced and heart-healthy diet.

One of the significant advantages lies in the emphasis on reducing sodium intake.

This cookbook encourage the use of herbs, spices, and other flavorful alternatives to salt, promoting a delicious culinary experience while lowering overall sodium consumption. This approach is instrumental in preventing hypertension and mitigating its effects on cardiovascular health.

Moreover, this cookbook contribute to weight management, a crucial factor in blood pressure control. The recommended recipes often emphasize portion control and include foods that support weight loss or maintenance.

By adopting the principles outlined in these cookbooks, individuals can make sustainable lifestyle changes that lead to improved overall health, reduced risk of heart-related complications, and enhanced well-being.

Tips for High Blood Pressure Cookbook

Emphasize whole, unprocessed foods: Encourage the use of fresh fruits, vegetables, whole grains, lean proteins, and healthy fats in recipes. These ingredients are rich in nutrients and fiber, which promote heart health and help lower blood pressure.

Reduce sodium: Provide tips for reducing sodium intake by using herbs, spices, and other flavor-enhancing ingredients instead of salt. Educate readers about reading food labels and choosing low-sodium alternatives.

Optimize cooking methods: Promote cooking techniques that retain nutrients and minimize the use of unhealthy fats. Encourage methods such as steaming, grilling, baking, and sautéing with heart-healthy oils like olive oil.

Focus on portion control: Offer guidance on appropriate portion sizes to help individuals manage calorie intake and maintain a healthy weight. Include tips for measuring portions and practicing mindful eating habits.

Include potassium-rich foods: Highlight ingredients high in potassium, such as bananas, spinach, avocado, and sweet potatoes, as they help counteract the effects of sodium on blood pressure.

Provide practical meal plans: Offer sample meal plans and recipes that showcase a balanced, heart-healthy diet. Include options for breakfast, lunch, dinner, and snacks to make meal planning easier for readers.

By incorporating these tips into this high blood pressure cookbook, individuals can learn how to make delicious and nutritious meals that support their cardiovascular health and overall well-being.

Guidelines of High Blood Pressure Cookbook

Nutrient-Rich Ingredients: Prioritize recipes that incorporate nutrient-dense foods, such as fruits, vegetables, whole grains, lean proteins, and sources of healthy fats like avocados and nuts.

Sodium Awareness: Emphasize the importance of reducing sodium intake. Provide alternatives to salt, encourage the use of herbs, spices, and low-sodium condiments, and educate readers on reading labels for hidden sources of sodium.

Balanced Macronutrients: Ensure a balance of carbohydrates, proteins, and fats in recipes to support overall health. Promote the use of heart-healthy fats, like those found in olive oil and fatty fish.

Portion Control: Guide individuals on appropriate portion sizes to help manage calorie intake and maintain a healthy weight. This is crucial for blood pressure management.

Hydration: Encourage an adequate intake of water and other hydrating beverages while minimizing the consumption of sugary drinks and excessive caffeine.

Mindful Eating: Promote mindful eating habits, such as slowing down during meals, savoring flavors, and recognizing hunger and fullness cues.

Limit Processed Foods: Minimize the inclusion of processed and packaged foods, which often contain high levels of sodium and unhealthy fats. Focus on whole, real foods.

Variety and Color: Encourage a diverse range of colorful fruits and vegetables to ensure a broad spectrum of nutrients and antioxidants.

Causes of High Blood Pressure

High blood pressure, or hypertension, can result from a combination of genetic, lifestyle, and environmental factors.

One primary cause is **Genetics**: Individuals with a family history of hypertension are more likely to develop high blood pressure themselves. Genetic factors can influence how the body regulates fluids and sodium, impacting blood pressure.

Unhealthy Lifestyle Habits contribute significantly to high blood pressure. Poor diet, especially one high in sodium and low in potassium-rich foods, can lead to hypertension. Lack of physical activity and sedentary behavior also contribute to elevated blood pressure.

Obesity is a significant risk factor for hypertension. Excess body weight puts a strain on the heart, requiring it to pump blood with more force, leading to increased pressure in the arteries.

Age is another factor, as blood vessels naturally lose flexibility and become stiffer over time. This can result in a rise in blood pressure, especially if unhealthy lifestyle habits are present.

Chronic Conditions such as kidney disease, diabetes, and sleep apnea can contribute to hypertension. These conditions can disrupt the body's natural blood pressure regulation mechanisms.

Stress and Mental Health: Chronic stress and certain mental health conditions can temporarily elevate blood pressure. While not a direct cause, long-term stress may contribute to unhealthy lifestyle choices that increase the risk of hypertension.

Understanding and addressing these causes are crucial for preventing and managing high blood pressure through lifestyle modifications and, if necessary, medical intervention.

Types of High blood Pressure Cookbook

There are two main types of high blood pressure, each with distinct characteristics: **Primary** (essential) hypertension and **Secondary** hypertension.

Primary Hypertension:

Primary hypertension is the most common type, accounting for about 90-95% of cases. It develops gradually over time and has no identifiable cause.

Multiple factors contribute to primary hypertension, including genetics, age, and lifestyle choices such as diet, physical activity, and stress. This type often develops over the years and is associated with aging.

Secondary Hypertension:

Secondary hypertension is less common and arises suddenly. It is often caused by an underlying condition that affects the kidneys, arteries, heart, or endocrine system.

Conditions such as kidney disease, hormonal disorders, obstructive sleep apnea, and certain medications can lead to secondary hypertension. Treating the underlying cause can sometimes normalize blood pressure levels.

In both types, high blood pressure can lead to serious health complications if left uncontrolled. Regular monitoring, lifestyle modifications, and, in some cases, medication are key components of managing hypertension.

Understanding the specific type of high blood pressure is crucial for developing an effective treatment plan tailored to the individual's needs.

Symptoms of High Blood Pressure

High blood pressure, also known as **hypertension**, is often referred to as the "silent killer" because it typically presents with no obvious symptoms in its early stages. However, as the condition progresses, some individuals may experience symptoms related to the effects of elevated blood pressure on the body.

Headaches: Persistent headaches, especially at the back of the head, can be a symptom of hypertension. However, headaches alone are not specific to high blood pressure and can have various causes.

Vision Problems: Blurred or impaired vision can occur when high blood pressure affects the blood vessels in the eyes. This can lead to retinopathy, a condition that damages the retina.

Chest Pain and Irregular Heartbeat: Severe hypertension can strain the heart, leading to chest pain (angina) or an irregular heartbeat (arrhythmia).

Fatigue and Confusion: Persistent fatigue, difficulty concentrating, and feelings of confusion can be associated with poorly controlled hypertension affecting blood flow to the brain.

Shortness of Breath: Difficulty breathing or shortness of breath may occur if high blood pressure contributes to heart failure, a condition where the heart cannot pump blood effectively.

It's crucial to note that these symptoms are often indicative of advanced stages of hypertension.

Regular blood pressure monitoring is essential, as early detection and management are key to preventing serious complications associated with high blood pressure. Individuals with risk factors should have their blood pressure checked regularly, even in the absence of symptoms.

High blood pressure, or **hypertension**, is influenced by a combination of genetic, lifestyle, and environmental factors. Several risk factors increase the likelihood of developing this condition:

Age: The risk of hypertension increases with age. As blood vessels lose elasticity over time, blood pressure tends to rise.

Family History: Individuals with a family history of hypertension are at a higher risk. Genetic factors play a role in how the body regulates blood pressure.

Race/Ethnicity: Certain ethnic groups, such as African Americans, are more prone to developing hypertension. They often experience it earlier in life and have higher average blood pressure levels.

Obesity: Being overweight or obese significantly increases the risk of hypertension. Excess weight requires the heart to pump blood with more force, leading to elevated blood pressure.

Unhealthy Lifestyle Habits: Poor diet, high sodium intake, lack of physical activity, excessive alcohol consumption, and smoking contribute to hypertension. These modifiable risk factors can be addressed through lifestyle changes.

Chronic Conditions: Conditions like diabetes, kidney disease, and sleep apnea are associated with an increased risk of hypertension. Managing these conditions is crucial for blood pressure control.

Stress: While not a direct cause, chronic stress can contribute to unhealthy lifestyle habits that may lead to hypertension.

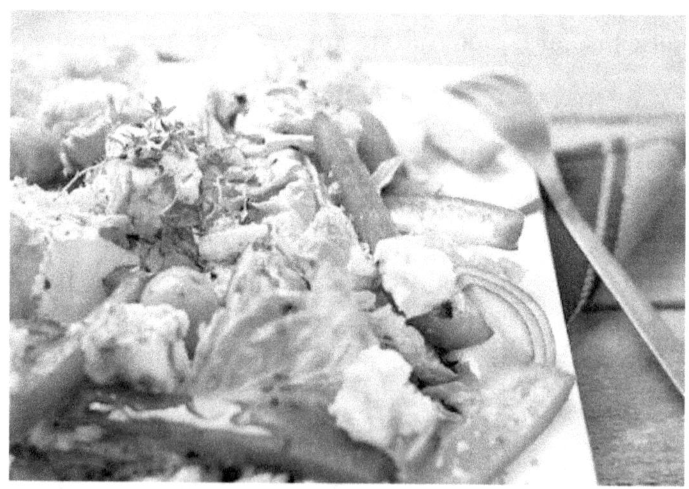

CHAPTER TWO

1: Grilled Salmon with Herb Quinoa

Ingredients:

- 4 salmon fillets
- 1 cup quinoa
- 2 cups vegetable broth
- 1 tablespoon olive oil
- 2 cloves garlic, minced
- 1 tablespoon chopped fresh herbs (such as parsley, dill, or basil)
- Salt and pepper to taste

Instructions:

- Preheat grill to medium-high heat.
- Rinse quinoa under cold water. In a saucepan, bring vegetable broth to a boil.
- Add quinoa, reduce heat to low, cover, and simmer for 15-20 minutes until liquid is absorbed.

- ➢ Meanwhile, brush salmon fillets with olive oil and season with minced garlic, chopped herbs, salt, and pepper.
- ➢ Grill salmon for 4-5 minutes per side until cooked through.
- ➢ Fluff quinoa with a fork and serve with grilled salmon.

Health Benefits:

- ➢ Salmon is rich in omega-3 fatty acids, which can help lower blood pressure and reduce inflammation.
- ➢ Quinoa is a whole grain high in fiber and protein, promoting heart health and aiding in blood pressure regulation.

Preparation Time: 25 minutes

2: Mediterranean Chickpea Salad

Ingredients:

- ➢ 2 cups canned chickpeas, drained and rinsed
- ➢ 1 cup cherry tomatoes, halved
- ➢ 1 cucumber, diced
- ➢ 1/2 red onion, finely chopped

- ➤ 1/4 cup feta cheese, crumbled
- ➤ 2 tablespoons extra-virgin olive oil
- ➤ 1 tablespoon red wine vinegar
- ➤ 1 teaspoon dried oregano
- ➤ Salt and pepper to taste

Instructions:

- ➤ In a large bowl, combine chickpeas, cherry tomatoes, cucumber, red onion, and feta cheese.
- ➤ In a small bowl, whisk together olive oil, red wine vinegar, dried oregano, salt, and pepper.
- ➤ Pour the dressing over the salad and toss to combine.
- ➤ Refrigerate for at least 30 minutes before serving.

Health Benefits:

- ➤ Chickpeas are high in potassium and fiber, supporting blood pressure regulation.
- ➤ Olive oil provides heart-healthy monounsaturated fats.

Preparation Time: 15 minutes

3: Spinach and Mushroom Stuffed Chicken Breast

Ingredients:

- 4 boneless, skinless chicken breasts
- 2 cups fresh spinach, chopped
- 1 cup mushrooms, sliced
- 1/2 cup low-fat mozzarella cheese, shredded
- 2 cloves garlic, minced
- 1 teaspoon olive oil
- 1 teaspoon dried thyme
- Salt and pepper to taste

Instructions:

- Preheat oven to 375°F (190°C).
- In a skillet, heat olive oil over medium heat. Add garlic, mushrooms, and spinach; sauté until vegetables are tender.
- Butterfly chicken breasts and stuff with sautéed spinach and mushrooms. Season with thyme, salt, and pepper.

- Place stuffed chicken breasts in a baking dish and bake for 25-30 minutes until chicken is cooked through.
- Sprinkle mozzarella cheese over the chicken during the last 5 minutes of baking.

Health Benefits:

- Spinach is rich in potassium, magnesium, and folate, all beneficial for blood pressure.
- Chicken is a lean protein source.

Preparation Time: 40 minutes

4: Quinoa and Black Bean Bowl

Ingredients:

- 1 cup quinoa, rinsed
- 2 cups vegetable broth
- 1 can black beans, drained and rinsed
- 1 cup corn kernels (fresh or frozen)
- 1 red bell pepper, diced
- 1 avocado, sliced
- 1 lime, juiced
- 2 tablespoons cilantro, chopped

- ➢ Salt and pepper to taste

Instructions:

- ➢ In a saucepan, bring vegetable broth to a boil. Add quinoa, reduce heat to low, cover, and simmer for 15-20 minutes until liquid is absorbed.
- ➢ In a large bowl, combine cooked quinoa, black beans, corn, red bell pepper, avocado, lime juice, cilantro, salt, and pepper.
- ➢ Toss the ingredients until well combined.
- ➢ Serve in bowls, and garnish with additional lime wedges if desired.

Health Benefits:

- ➢ Quinoa is a whole grain with potassium and magnesium, supporting blood pressure regulation.
- ➢ Black beans are high in fiber and protein, promoting heart health.

Preparation Time: 30 minutes

5: Roasted Vegetable and Lentil Salad

Ingredients:

- ➢ 1 cup dried green lentils, rinsed

- 3 cups mixed vegetables (zucchini, bell peppers, cherry tomatoes), chopped
- 2 tablespoons olive oil
- 2 cloves garlic, minced
- 1 teaspoon dried rosemary
- Salt and pepper to taste
- 1/4 cup balsamic vinegar
- 2 tablespoons fresh basil, chopped

Instructions:

- Preheat oven to 400°F (200°C).
- In a pot, cook lentils according to package instructions.
- In a large bowl, toss chopped vegetables with olive oil, garlic, rosemary, salt, and pepper.
- Spread the vegetables on a baking sheet and roast for 20-25 minutes until golden brown.
- In a bowl, combine cooked lentils, roasted vegetables, balsamic vinegar, and fresh basil. Toss to combine.

Health Benefits:

➢ Lentils are rich in potassium and fiber, supporting heart health.

➢ Vegetables provide antioxidants and essential nutrients.

Preparation Time: 40 minutes

6: Turkey and Vegetable Stir-Fry

Ingredients:

➢ 1 pound lean ground turkey

➢ 2 cups broccoli florets

➢ 1 red bell pepper, sliced

➢ 1 cup snap peas, trimmed

➢ 2 carrots, julienned

➢ 3 tablespoons low-sodium soy sauce

➢ 1 tablespoon sesame oil

➢ 2 teaspoons ginger, minced

➢ 2 cloves garlic, minced

➢ 1 tablespoon rice vinegar

➢ 1 tablespoon honey

➢ Brown rice or quinoa (optional, for serving)

Instructions:

> - In a large skillet, cook ground turkey over medium heat until browned.
> - Add broccoli, bell pepper, snap peas, and carrots to the skillet. Stir-fry for 5-7 minutes until vegetables are tender-crisp.
> - In a small bowl, whisk together soy sauce, sesame oil, ginger, garlic, rice vinegar, and honey.
> - Pour the sauce over the turkey and vegetables, tossing to coat evenly.
> - Serve the stir-fry over brown rice or quinoa if desired.

Health Benefits:

> - Lean ground turkey is a good source of protein.
> - Vegetables provide essential vitamins and minerals.

Preparation Time: 25 minutes

7: Lentil and Vegetable Soup

Ingredients:

> - 1 cup dried green or brown lentils, rinsed
> - 1 onion, chopped

- 2 carrots, diced
- 2 celery stalks, chopped
- 3 cloves garlic, minced
- 1 can diced tomatoes (low-sodium)
- 6 cups vegetable broth (low-sodium)
- 1 teaspoon ground cumin
- 1 teaspoon paprika
- 1/2 teaspoon dried thyme
- Salt and pepper to taste
- Fresh parsley, chopped (for garnish)

Instructions:

- In a large pot, combine lentils, onion, carrots, celery, garlic, diced tomatoes, vegetable broth, cumin, paprika, thyme, salt, and pepper.
- Bring the mixture to a boil, then reduce the heat to low and simmer for 25-30 minutes or until lentils are tender.
- Adjust seasoning as needed.
- Serve hot, garnished with fresh parsley.

Health Benefits:

- Lentils are rich in fiber, potassium, and folate.

- ➢ Vegetables contribute essential nutrients and antioxidants.

Preparation Time: 40 minutes

8: Baked Cod with Lemon and Herbs

Ingredients:

- ➢ 4 cod fillets
- ➢ 2 tablespoons olive oil
- ➢ 2 tablespoons fresh lemon juice
- ➢ 1 teaspoon dried thyme
- ➢ 1 teaspoon dried rosemary
- ➢ 1 teaspoon paprika
- ➢ Salt and pepper to taste
- ➢ Fresh parsley, chopped (for garnish)

Instructions:

- ➢ Preheat oven to 400°F (200°C).
- ➢ Place cod fillets on a baking sheet lined with parchment paper.
- ➢ In a small bowl, mix olive oil, lemon juice, thyme, rosemary, paprika, salt, and pepper.
- ➢ Brush the mixture over the cod fillets.

➢ Bake for 15-20 minutes or until the fish flakes easily with a fork.

➢ Garnish with fresh parsley before serving.

Health Benefits:

➢ Cod is a lean protein source.

➢ Olive oil provides heart-healthy monounsaturated fats.

Preparation Time: 25 minutes

9: Quinoa and Vegetable Stuffed Peppers

Ingredients:

➢ 1 cup quinoa, cooked

➢ 4 bell peppers, halved and seeds removed

➢ 1 can black beans, drained and rinsed

➢ 1 cup corn kernels (fresh or frozen)

➢ 1 cup cherry tomatoes, halved

➢ 1 cup spinach, chopped

➢ 1 teaspoon ground cumin

➢ 1 teaspoon chili powder

➢ Salt and pepper to taste

➢ 1 cup shredded cheddar cheese (optional)

Instructions:

> Preheat oven to 375°F (190°C).
> In a large bowl, mix together cooked quinoa, black beans, corn, cherry tomatoes, spinach, cumin, chili powder, salt, and pepper.
> Fill each bell pepper half with the quinoa mixture.
> Place stuffed peppers in a baking dish. If desired, sprinkle shredded cheddar cheese on top.
> Bake for 25-30 minutes or until peppers are tender.

Health Benefits:

> Quinoa provides protein and essential nutrients.
> Vegetables contribute fiber, vitamins, and minerals.

Preparation Time: 40 minutes

10: Greek Yogurt Parfait with Berries

Ingredients:

> 1 cup Greek yogurt (low-fat or non-fat)
> 1 cup mixed berries (strawberries, blueberries, raspberries)
> 1/4 cup granola
> 1 tablespoon honey

➢ Fresh mint leaves (for garnish)

Instructions:

➢ In a glass or bowl, layer Greek yogurt, mixed berries, and granola.
➢ Drizzle honey over the top.
➢ Garnish with fresh mint leaves.

Health Benefits:

➢ Greek yogurt is a good source of protein and calcium.
➢ Berries are rich in antioxidants and contribute to heart health.

Preparation Time: 5 minutes

11: Vegetable and Bean Chili

Ingredients:

➢ 1 tablespoon olive oil
➢ 1 onion, chopped
➢ 2 cloves garlic, minced
➢ 1 bell pepper, diced
➢ 1 zucchini, diced
➢ 1 carrot, diced
➢ 1 can diced tomatoes (low-sodium)

- ➢ 1 can kidney beans, drained and rinsed

- ➢ 1 can black beans, drained and rinsed

- ➢ 2 cups vegetable broth (low-sodium)

- ➢ 1 tablespoon chili powder

- ➢ 1 teaspoon ground cumin

- ➢ Salt and pepper to taste

- ➢ Fresh cilantro, chopped (for garnish)

Instructions:

- ➢ In a large pot, heat olive oil over medium heat. Add onion and garlic, sauté until softened.

- ➢ Add bell pepper, zucchini, and carrot, cook for 5 minutes.

- ➢ Stir in diced tomatoes, kidney beans, black beans, vegetable broth, chili powder, cumin, salt, and pepper.

- ➢ Bring to a boil, then reduce heat and simmer for 20-25 minutes.

- ➢ Adjust seasoning as needed. Serve hot, garnished with fresh cilantro.

Health Benefits:

> ➢ Beans are high in fiber and protein, aiding in blood pressure regulation.
> ➢ Vegetables provide essential nutrients and antioxidants.

Preparation Time: 35 minutes

12: Oven-Roasted Vegetables

Ingredients:

> ➢ Assorted vegetables (such as bell peppers, zucchini, eggplant, cherry tomatoes)
> ➢ 2 tablespoons olive oil
> ➢ 2 cloves garlic, minced
> ➢ 1 teaspoon dried herbs (such as thyme, rosemary, or oregano)
> ➢ Salt and pepper to taste
> ➢ Fresh parsley, chopped (for garnish)

Instructions:

> ➢ Preheat oven to 400°F (200°C).
> ➢ Cut vegetables into bite-sized pieces and place them on a baking sheet lined with parchment paper.

- In a small bowl, mix together olive oil, minced garlic, dried herbs, salt, and pepper.
- Drizzle the olive oil mixture over the vegetables and toss to coat evenly.
- Roast in the oven for 20-25 minutes until vegetables are tender and slightly caramelized.
- Garnish with fresh parsley before serving.

Health Benefits:

- Vegetables are rich in potassium, fiber, and antioxidants, supporting heart health.

Preparation Time: 30 minutes

13: Tuna and White Bean Salad

Ingredients:

- 2 cans tuna, drained
- 1 can white beans (such as cannellini or navy beans), drained and rinsed
- 1 red onion, finely chopped
- 1 bell pepper, diced
- 1 cucumber, diced
- 1/4 cup Kalamata olives, sliced

- ➢ 2 tablespoons extra-virgin olive oil
- ➢ 1 tablespoon lemon juice
- ➢ 1 teaspoon Dijon mustard
- ➢ Salt and pepper to taste
- ➢ Fresh parsley, chopped (for garnish)

Instructions:

- ➢ In a large bowl, combine tuna, white beans, red onion, bell pepper, cucumber, and Kalamata olives.
- ➢ In a small bowl, whisk together olive oil, lemon juice, Dijon mustard, salt, and pepper.
- ➢ Pour the dressing over the tuna and bean mixture, tossing to coat evenly.
- ➢ Garnish with fresh parsley before serving.

Health Benefits:

- ➢ Tuna is a lean protein source.
- ➢ White beans are high in fiber and potassium.

Preparation Time: 15 minutes

14: Lemon Garlic Shrimp with Asparagus

Ingredients:

- ➢ 1-pound shrimp, peeled and deveined

- ➢ 1 bunch asparagus, trimmed
- ➢ 2 tablespoons olive oil
- ➢ 3 cloves garlic, minced
- ➢ 1 lemon, zest and juice
- ➢ Salt and pepper to taste
- ➢ Fresh parsley, chopped (for garnish)

Instructions:

- ➢ Preheat oven to 400°F (200°C).
- ➢ Place shrimp and asparagus on a baking sheet lined with parchment paper.
- ➢ In a small bowl, whisk together olive oil, minced garlic, lemon zest, lemon juice, salt, and pepper.
- ➢ Drizzle the olive oil mixture over the shrimp and asparagus, tossing to coat evenly.
- ➢ Roast in the oven for 8-10 minutes until shrimp are pink and cooked through.
- ➢ Garnish with fresh parsley before serving.

Health Benefits:

- ➢ Shrimp is a low-calorie source of protein.
- ➢ Asparagus is high in potassium and folate.

Preparation Time: 20 minutes

15: Avocado and Tomato Salad

Ingredients:

> - 2 avocados, diced
> - 2 cups cherry tomatoes, halved
> - 1/4 red onion, thinly sliced
> - 2 tablespoons fresh basil, chopped
> - 1 tablespoon extra-virgin olive oil
> - 1 tablespoon balsamic vinegar
> - Salt and pepper to taste

Instructions:

> - In a large bowl, combine diced avocados, cherry tomatoes, red onion, and chopped basil.
> - In a small bowl, whisk together olive oil, balsamic vinegar, salt, and pepper.
> - Pour the dressing over the avocado and tomato mixture, tossing to coat evenly.
> - Serve immediately.

Health Benefits:

> - Avocado is rich in heart-healthy monounsaturated fats.

> Tomatoes are high in potassium and antioxidants.

Preparation Time: 10 minutes

16: Eggplant and Tomato Ratatouille

Ingredients:

- 1 eggplant, diced
- 2 zucchinis, diced
- 1 onion, diced
- 2 bell peppers, diced
- 3 cloves garlic, minced
- 1 can diced tomatoes (low-sodium)
- 2 tablespoons olive oil
- 1 teaspoon dried thyme
- 1 teaspoon dried oregano
- Salt and pepper to taste
- Fresh basil, chopped (for garnish)

Instructions:

- In a large skillet, heat olive oil over medium heat. Add diced onion and minced garlic, sauté until softened.

- ➢ Add diced eggplant, zucchinis, bell peppers, dried thyme, dried oregano, salt, and pepper. Cook for 8-10 minutes until vegetables are tender.
- ➢ Stir in diced tomatoes and simmer for 5 minutes.
- ➢ Adjust seasoning as needed. Serve hot, garnished with fresh basil.

Health Benefits:

- ➢ Eggplant is rich in fiber and antioxidants.
- ➢ Zucchini and bell peppers provide essential nutrients and vitamins.

Preparation Time: 30 minutes

17: Chicken and Vegetable Stir-Fry

Ingredients:

- ➢ 1 pound boneless, skinless chicken breasts, thinly sliced
- ➢ 2 cups mixed vegetables (bell peppers, broccoli, carrots), sliced
- ➢ 2 cloves garlic, minced
- ➢ 1 tablespoon ginger, minced
- ➢ 2 tablespoons low-sodium soy sauce

- ➢ 1 tablespoon hoisin sauce

- ➢ 1 teaspoon sesame oil

- ➢ 2 tablespoons olive oil

- ➢ Salt and pepper to taste

- ➢ Cooked brown rice (optional, for serving)

Instructions:

- ➢ In a large skillet or wok, heat olive oil over medium-high heat.

- ➢ Add minced garlic and ginger, and sauté until fragrant.

- ➢ Add sliced chicken breasts to the skillet and cook until browned and cooked through.

- ➢ Add mixed vegetables and stir-fry for 4-5 minutes until tender-crisp.

- ➢ In a small bowl, whisk together soy sauce, hoisin sauce, and sesame oil. Pour over the chicken and vegetables, tossing to coat.

- ➢ Serve hot over cooked brown rice if desired.

Health Benefits:

- ➢ Lean chicken breast provides protein.

> Mixed vegetables are rich in vitamins, minerals, and
> fiber.

Preparation Time: 30 minutes

18: Tomato Basil Bruschetta

Ingredients:

- 4 large tomatoes, diced
- 2 cloves garlic, minced
- 1/4 cup fresh basil, chopped
- 2 tablespoons extra-virgin olive oil
- 1 tablespoon balsamic vinegar
- Salt and pepper to taste
- Whole grain baguette, sliced and toasted

Instructions:

- In a bowl, combine diced tomatoes, minced garlic, chopped basil, olive oil, balsamic vinegar, salt, and pepper.
- Mix well to combine and let sit for 10-15 minutes to allow flavors to meld.
- Spoon tomato mixture onto toasted whole grain baguette slices.

➢ Serve immediately as an appetizer or snack.

Health Benefits:

➢ Tomatoes are rich in lycopene, which may help lower blood pressure.

➢ Olive oil provides heart-healthy monounsaturated fats.

Preparation Time: 15 minutes

19: Lentil and Vegetable Curry

Ingredients:

➢ 1 cup dried green lentils, rinsed

➢ 1 onion, chopped

➢ 2 cloves garlic, minced

➢ 1 tablespoon ginger, minced

➢ 1 tablespoon curry powder

➢ 1 teaspoon ground cumin

➢ 1 teaspoon ground coriander

➢ 1 can coconut milk (light)

➢ 2 cups mixed vegetables (bell peppers, carrots, peas)

➢ Salt and pepper to taste

➢ Fresh cilantro, chopped (for garnish)

➢ Cooked brown rice (optional, for serving)

Instructions:

➢ In a large pot, sauté chopped onion, minced garlic, and minced ginger until softened.
➢ Add curry powder, ground cumin, and ground coriander, and cook for 1-2 minutes until fragrant.
➢ Stir in rinsed lentils and mixed vegetables.
➢ Pour in coconut milk and enough water to cover the ingredients. Bring to a boil, then reduce heat to low and simmer for 20-25 minutes until lentils are tender.
➢ Season with salt and pepper to taste.
➢ Serve hot over cooked brown rice, garnished with chopped cilantro.

Health Benefits:

➢ Lentils are rich in fiber and protein.
➢ Coconut milk provides healthy fats and adds creaminess to the curry.

Preparation Time: 40 minutes

20: Turkey and Bean Chili

Ingredients:

- ➢ 1 pound lean ground turkey
- ➢ 1 onion, chopped
- ➢ 2 cloves garlic, minced
- ➢ 1 bell pepper, diced
- ➢ 1 can diced tomatoes (low-sodium)
- ➢ 1 can kidney beans, drained and rinsed
- ➢ 1 can black beans, drained and rinsed
- ➢ 2 cups vegetable broth (low-sodium)
- ➢ 2 tablespoons chili powder
- ➢ 1 teaspoon ground cumin
- ➢ Salt and pepper to taste
- ➢ Fresh cilantro, chopped (for garnish)

Instructions:

- ➢ In a large pot, cook lean ground turkey over medium heat until browned.
- ➢ Add chopped onion, minced garlic, and diced bell pepper to the pot. Sauté until vegetables are softened.
- ➢ Stir in diced tomatoes, kidney beans, black beans, vegetable broth, chili powder, and ground cumin.

- ➢ Bring the chili to a simmer, then reduce heat to low and cook for 20-25 minutes, stirring occasionally.
- ➢ Season with salt and pepper to taste.
- ➢ Serve hot, garnished with chopped cilantro.

Health Benefits:

- ➢ Lean ground turkey provides protein.
- ➢ Beans are high in fiber and potassium, promoting heart health.

Preparation Time: 40 minutes

21: Eggplant and Chickpea Curry

Ingredients:

- ➢ 1 large eggplant, diced
- ➢ 1 can chickpeas, drained and rinsed
- ➢ 1 onion, chopped
- ➢ 2 cloves garlic, minced
- ➢ 1 tablespoon ginger, minced
- ➢ 1 tablespoon curry powder
- ➢ 1 teaspoon ground cumin
- ➢ 1 teaspoon ground coriander
- ➢ 1 can diced tomatoes (low-sodium)

- ➢ 1 can coconut milk (light)
- ➢ Salt and pepper to taste
- ➢ Fresh cilantro, chopped (for garnish)
- ➢ Cooked brown rice (optional, for serving)

Instructions:

- ➢ In a large skillet, sauté chopped onion, minced garlic, and minced ginger until softened.
- ➢ Add diced eggplant to the skillet and cook until slightly softened.
- ➢ Stir in curry powder, ground cumin, and ground coriander, and cook for 1-2 minutes until fragrant.
- ➢ Add drained chickpeas, diced tomatoes, and coconut milk to the skillet. Bring to a simmer and cook for 15-20 minutes until eggplant is tender.
- ➢ Season with salt and pepper to taste.
- ➢ Serve hot over cooked brown rice, garnished with chopped cilantro.

Health Benefits:

- ➢ Eggplant is low in calories and rich in fiber and antioxidants.
- ➢ Chickpeas provide protein and fiber.

Preparation Time: 40 minutes

22: Grilled Salmon with Lemon and Herbs

Ingredients:

- ➢ 4 salmon fillets
- ➢ 2 tablespoons olive oil
- ➢ 1 lemon (juiced and zested)
- ➢ 2 cloves garlic (minced)
- ➢ 1 teaspoon dried herbs (such as thyme or rosemary)
- ➢ Salt and pepper to taste

Instructions:

- ➢ Preheat the grill.
- ➢ In a bowl, mix olive oil, lemon juice, lemon zest, minced garlic, dried herbs, salt, and pepper.
- ➢ Brush the salmon fillets with the mixture.
- ➢ Grill the salmon for 4-5 minutes on each side or until cooked through.
- ➢ Serve with a side of steamed vegetables.

Health Benefits:

- ➢ Salmon is rich in omega-3 fatty acids, which have been associated with lower blood pressure.

Preparation Time: 20 minutes

23: Quinoa Salad with Avocado and Cherry Tomatoes

Ingredients:

- 1 cup quinoa (cooked)
- 1 avocado (diced)
- 1 cup cherry tomatoes (halved)
- 1/4 cup red onion (finely chopped)
- 2 tablespoons olive oil
- 2 tablespoons balsamic vinegar
- Salt and pepper to taste

Instructions:

- In a bowl, combine quinoa, diced avocado, cherry tomatoes, and red onion.
- In a small bowl, whisk together olive oil, balsamic vinegar, salt, and pepper.
- Pour the dressing over the quinoa mixture and toss gently.
- Chill before serving.

Health Benefits:

> Quinoa is a whole grain that is high in fiber and may contribute to lower blood pressure.

Preparation Time: 25 minutes

24: Garlic and Herb Roasted Sweet Potatoes

Ingredients:

> 3 sweet potatoes (peeled and cubed)
> 2 tablespoons olive oil
> 3 cloves garlic (minced)
> 1 teaspoon dried herbs (such as thyme or rosemary)
> Salt and pepper to taste

Instructions:

> Preheat the oven to 400°F (200°C).
> In a bowl, toss sweet potato cubes with olive oil, minced garlic, dried herbs, salt, and pepper.
> Spread the sweet potatoes on a baking sheet in a single layer.
> Roast for 25-30 minutes or until tender and golden.

Health Benefits:

> Sweet potatoes are rich in potassium, which may help regulate blood pressure.

Preparation Time: 35 minutes

25: Mediterranean Chickpea Salad

Ingredients:

> 1 can (15 oz) chickpeas (rinsed and drained)
> 1 cucumber (diced)
> 1 cup cherry tomatoes (halved)
> 1/2 cup feta cheese (crumbled)
> 1/4 cup red onion (finely chopped)
> 2 tablespoons olive oil
> 2 tablespoons lemon juice
> 1 teaspoon dried oregano
> Salt and pepper to taste

Instructions:

> In a large bowl, combine chickpeas, cucumber, cherry tomatoes, feta cheese, and red onion.
> In a small bowl, whisk together olive oil, lemon juice, dried oregano, salt, and pepper.

- ➢ Pour the dressing over the salad and toss gently.
- ➢ Refrigerate for at least 30 minutes before serving.

Health Benefits:

- ➢ Chickpeas are high in fiber and may help support heart health.

Preparation Time: 20 minutes

26: Spinach and Berry Smoothie

Ingredients:

- ➢ 2 cups fresh spinach
- ➢ 1 cup mixed berries (strawberries, blueberries, raspberries)
- ➢ 1 banana
- ➢ 1 cup low-fat yogurt
- ➢ 1/2 cup almond milk
- ➢ 1 tablespoon chia seeds

Instructions:

- ➢ Blend spinach, berries, banana, yogurt, and almond milk until smooth.
- ➢ Stir in chia seeds.
- ➢ Pour into a glass and enjoy immediately.

Health Benefits:

> Berries are rich in antioxidants, and spinach provides essential nutrients that support heart health.

Preparation Time: 10 minutes

27: Lentil and Vegetable Stir-Fry

Ingredients:

> 1 cup dry lentils (cooked)
> 2 cups mixed vegetables (broccoli, bell peppers, snap peas)
> 2 tablespoons low-sodium soy sauce
> 1 tablespoon sesame oil
> 2 cloves garlic (minced)
> 1 teaspoon ginger (grated)
> 1 tablespoon olive oil
> Instructions:
> In a wok or large pan, heat olive oil over medium heat.
> Add minced garlic and grated ginger, sauté for 1 minute.
> Add mixed vegetables and stir-fry until tender-crisp.

➢ Stir in cooked lentils, soy sauce, and sesame oil. Cook for an additional 2-3 minutes.

➢ Serve over brown rice or quinoa.

Health Benefits:

➢ Lentils are rich in fiber and protein, contributing to heart health.

Preparation Time: 30 minutes

28: Baked Herb-Crusted Chicken

Ingredients:

➢ 4 boneless, skinless chicken breasts

➢ 2 tablespoons olive oil

➢ 1 tablespoon dried Italian herbs (basil, oregano, thyme)

➢ 2 cloves garlic (minced)

➢ Salt and pepper to taste

Instructions:

➢ Preheat the oven to 375°F (190°C).

➢ Rub chicken breasts with olive oil and minced garlic.

➢ Sprinkle dried herbs, salt, and pepper evenly over the chicken.

> Bake for 25-30 minutes or until the chicken is cooked through.

Health Benefits:

> Lean chicken is a good source of protein and a healthier alternative to red meat.

Preparation Time: 35 minutes

29: Greek Yogurt Parfait

Ingredients:

> 1 cup plain Greek yogurt
> 1/2 cup granola (low in added sugar)
> 1/2 cup mixed berries (blueberries, strawberries)
> 1 tablespoon honey

Instructions:

> In a glass or bowl, layer Greek yogurt, granola, and mixed berries.
> Drizzle honey over the top.
> Repeat the layers as desired.
> Serve chilled.

Health Benefits:

➢ Greek yogurt is a good source of protein and probiotics, supporting heart health.

Preparation Time: 10 minutes

30: Roasted Brussels Sprouts with Walnuts

Ingredients:

➢ 1 pound Brussels sprouts (trimmed and halved)
➢ 1/2 cup walnuts (chopped)
➢ 2 tablespoons olive oil
➢ 1 tablespoon balsamic vinegar
➢ Salt and pepper to taste

Instructions:

➢ Preheat the oven to 400°F (200°C).
➢ Toss Brussels sprouts and walnuts with olive oil, balsamic vinegar, salt, and pepper.
➢ Spread the mixture on a baking sheet.
➢ Roast for 20-25 minutes or until Brussels sprouts are golden and tender.

Health Benefits:

- Brussels sprouts are rich in fiber, vitamins, and minerals that contribute to heart health.

Preparation Time: 30 minutes

31: Spinach and Feta Stuffed Chicken Breast

Ingredients:

- 4 boneless, skinless chicken breasts
- 2 cups fresh spinach (chopped)
- 1/2 cup feta cheese (crumbled)
- 2 tablespoons olive oil
- 1 teaspoon dried oregano
- Salt and pepper to taste

Instructions:

- Preheat the oven to 375°F (190°C).
- In a bowl, combine chopped spinach, crumbled feta, olive oil, dried oregano, salt, and pepper.
- Cut a pocket in each chicken breast and stuff with the spinach and feta mixture.
- Bake for 25-30 minutes or until the chicken is cooked through.

Health Benefits:

- ➢ Spinach is rich in potassium, and the lean chicken provides protein for heart health.

Preparation Time: 40 minutes

32: Quinoa and Black Bean Stuffed Peppers

Ingredients:

- ➢ 4 bell peppers (halved and seeds removed)
- ➢ 1 cup quinoa (cooked)
- ➢ 1 can (15 oz) black beans (rinsed and drained)
- ➢ 1 cup corn kernels (fresh or frozen)
- ➢ 1 cup salsa
- ➢ 1 teaspoon cumin
- ➢ 1/2 teaspoon chili powder
- ➢ 1/2 cup shredded low-fat cheese

Instructions:

- ➢ Preheat the oven to 375°F (190°C).
- ➢ In a bowl, mix cooked quinoa, black beans, corn, salsa, cumin, and chili powder.
- ➢ Spoon the mixture into the halved bell peppers.
- ➢ Top with shredded cheese.

> Bake for 25-30 minutes or until the peppers are tender.

Health Benefits:

> Quinoa and black beans provide a combination of fiber and protein for heart health.

Preparation Time: 45 minutes

33: Lemon Garlic Shrimp Stir-Fry

Ingredients:

> 1 pound shrimp (peeled and deveined)
> 2 cups broccoli florets
> 1 bell pepper (sliced)
> 3 tablespoons soy sauce (low-sodium)
> 2 tablespoons olive oil
> 2 cloves garlic (minced)
> 1 teaspoon ginger (grated)
> Juice of 1 lemon

Instructions:

> In a wok or large pan, heat olive oil over medium heat.

➤ Add minced garlic and grated ginger, sauté for 1 minute.

➤ Add shrimp and stir-fry until pink.

➤ Add broccoli and bell pepper, continue to stir-fry until vegetables are tender.

➤ Pour soy sauce and lemon juice over the mixture, toss to combine.

Health Benefits:

➤ Shrimp is a low-calorie protein source, and vegetables provide essential nutrients for heart health.

Preparation Time: 20 minutes

34: Sweet Potato and Black Bean Chili

Ingredients:

➤ 2 sweet potatoes (peeled and diced)

➤ 1 can (15 oz) black beans (rinsed and drained)

➤ 1 can (14 oz) diced tomatoes (with juice)

➤ 1 onion (chopped)

➤ 2 cloves garlic (minced)

➤ 1 tablespoon olive oil

> 2 teaspoons chili powder

> 1 teaspoon cumin

> Salt and pepper to taste

Instructions:

> In a large pot, heat olive oil over medium heat.

> Add chopped onion and minced garlic, sauté until softened.

> Add diced sweet potatoes, black beans, diced tomatoes, chili powder, cumin, salt, and pepper.

> Simmer for 20-25 minutes or until sweet potatoes are tender.

Health Benefits:

> Sweet potatoes and black beans provide fiber, vitamins, and minerals beneficial for heart health.

Preparation Time: 40 minutes

35: Broccoli and Quinoa Casserole

Ingredients:

> 2 cups broccoli florets

> 1 cup quinoa (cooked)

> 1 cup shredded low-fat cheddar cheese

- ➢ 1/2 cup Greek yogurt

- ➢ 2 tablespoons whole wheat flour

- ➢ 2 cloves garlic (minced)

- ➢ Salt and pepper to taste

Instructions

- ➢ Preheat the oven to 375°F (190°C).

- ➢ Steam broccoli until slightly tender.

- ➢ In a bowl, mix cooked quinoa, steamed broccoli, shredded cheese, Greek yogurt, whole wheat flour, minced garlic, salt, and pepper.

- ➢ Transfer the mixture to a baking dish and bake for 25-30 minutes or until golden and bubbly.

Health Benefits:

- ➢ Broccoli is rich in antioxidants, and quinoa provides a good source of protein and fiber.

Preparation Time: 45 minutes

36: Turkey and Vegetable Skewers

Ingredients:

- ➢ 1 pound turkey breast (cut into chunks)

- ➢ 2 zucchini (sliced)

- ➢ 1 bell pepper (sliced)
- ➢ 1 red onion (sliced)
- ➢ 2 tablespoons olive oil
- ➢ 1 teaspoon dried Italian herbs
- ➢ Salt and pepper to taste

Instructions:

- ➢ Preheat the grill or grill pan.
- ➢ In a bowl, toss turkey chunks, zucchini, bell pepper, red onion, olive oil, dried Italian herbs, salt, and pepper.
- ➢ Thread the turkey and vegetables onto skewers.
- ➢ Grill for 10-15 minutes, turning occasionally, until turkey is cooked through and vegetables are tender.

Health Benefits:

- ➢ Lean turkey is a good source of protein, and vegetables add fiber and essential nutrients.

Preparation Time: 30 minutes

37: Cauliflower Rice Stir-Fry with Tofu

Ingredients:

- ➢ 1 block extra-firm tofu (pressed and cubed)

- ➤ 1 head cauliflower (riced)
- ➤ 2 cups mixed vegetables (carrots, peas, bell peppers)
- ➤ 3 tablespoons low-sodium soy sauce
- ➤ 1 tablespoon sesame oil
- ➤ 2 cloves garlic (minced)
- ➤ 1 teaspoon ginger (grated)
- ➤ 2 green onions (sliced)

Instructions:

- ➤ In a wok or large pan, heat sesame oil over medium heat.
- ➤ Add minced garlic and grated ginger, sauté for 1 minute.
- ➤ Add cubed tofu and stir-fry until golden.
- ➤ Add cauliflower rice and mixed vegetables, continue to stir-fry until vegetables are tender.
- ➤ Pour soy sauce over the mixture, toss to combine.
- ➤ Garnish with sliced green onions before serving.

Health Benefits:

- ➤ Cauliflower is a low-calorie, nutrient-rich alternative to rice, and tofu adds plant-based protein.

Preparation Time: 25 minutes

38: Berry and Almond Salad with Citrus Dressing

Ingredients:

> 4 cups mixed greens (spinach, arugula)
> 1 cup mixed berries (strawberries, blueberries, raspberries)
> 1/2 cup almonds (sliced)
> 1/4 cup feta cheese (optional)
> 2 tablespoons olive oil
> Juice of 1 orange
> 1 tablespoon honey
> Salt and pepper to taste

Instructions:

> In a large bowl, combine mixed greens, mixed berries, sliced almonds, and feta cheese.
> In a small bowl, whisk together olive oil, orange juice, honey, salt, and pepper.
> Drizzle the dressing over the salad and toss gently before serving.

Health Benefits:

> Berries are rich in antioxidants, and almonds provide healthy fats beneficial for heart health.

Preparation Time: 15 minutes

39: Cilantro Lime Shrimp and Avocado Salad

Ingredients:

> 1 pound shrimp (peeled and deveined)
> 2 avocados (diced)
> 1 cup cherry tomatoes (halved)
> 1/4 cup red onion (finely chopped)
> 1/4 cup fresh cilantro (chopped)
> Juice of 2 limes
> 2 tablespoons olive oil
> Salt and pepper to taste

Instructions:

> In a bowl, combine shrimp, diced avocados, cherry tomatoes, red onion, and cilantro.
> In a separate small bowl, whisk together lime juice, olive oil, salt, and pepper.
> Pour the dressing over the salad and toss gently.

➤ Serve chilled.

Health Benefits:

➤ Shrimp is a low-calorie protein source, and avocados provide heart-healthy monounsaturated fats.

Preparation Time: 20 minutes

40: Turkey and Vegetable Quinoa Bowl

Ingredients:

➤ 1 cup quinoa (cooked)

➤ 1 pound ground turkey

➤ 2 cups broccoli florets

➤ 1 bell pepper (sliced)

➤ 1 tablespoon olive oil

➤ 2 cloves garlic (minced)

➤ 2 teaspoons soy sauce (low-sodium)

➤ 1 teaspoon ground cumin

➤ Salt and pepper to taste

Instructions:

➤ In a large skillet, heat olive oil over medium heat.

➤ Add minced garlic and ground turkey, cook until browned.

- ➤ Add broccoli, bell pepper, soy sauce, ground cumin, salt, and pepper. Stir-fry until vegetables are tender.
- ➤ Serve the turkey and vegetable mixture over a bed of cooked quinoa.

Health Benefits:

- ➤ Turkey is a lean protein source, and quinoa adds fiber and essential nutrients.

Preparation Time: 30 minutes

CONCLUSION

This High Blood Pressure Cookbook serves as a comprehensive guide to not only satisfying your taste buds but also prioritizing your heart health.

By incorporating nutrient-rich ingredients, lean proteins, and heart-friendly choices, these recipes offer a delicious pathway to managing blood pressure and promoting overall well-being.

Remember, a heart-healthy diet is a crucial component of a balanced lifestyle, and these recipes provide a diverse range of flavors, textures, and nutritional benefits.

Whether you're a seasoned chef or a novice in the kitchen, this cookbook aims to inspire you to create meals that are not only good for your taste buds but also for your cardiovascular health.

As you embark on this culinary journey, consider consulting with healthcare professionals for personalized advice on managing blood pressure. Here's to delicious, heart-conscious meals that contribute to a healthier and happier you!